Essential Oils

For Beginners:

Aromatherapy and Essential Oils for Weight Loss, Natural Remedy, Stress Relief, Body Massage and Beauty

By

Brittany Samons

2

Table of Contents

Essential Oils For Beginners: Aromatherapy and
Essential Oils for Weight Loss, Natural Remedy, Stress
Relief, Body Massage and Beauty

By Brittany Samons

© Copyright 2014 Brittany Samons

First Published, 2014

Printed in the United States of America

Introduction

Essential oils are truly amazing and have great uses for the skin and the body as a whole. If you are looking into using essential oils for certain ailments and illnesses, then you better understand first the very nature and different aspects of this aromatic sensation. I say aromatherapy because essential oils are the main ingredients of performing aromatherapy and have proven to be very useful and healthy for anybody who decides to use them.

Have you had your aromatherapy session? It's actually quite refreshing and relaxing, not to mention recharging for the whole body and mind. You will have a choice of what kind of essential oils you can use and what specific problem areas you would like to target. If you have not tried one before then maybe this book will get you to think of taking a gander and have a taste.

Chapter 1. Aromatherapy Basics

Aromatherapy was first popularized since the late 1930's through a book by a French chemist Rene-Maurice Gattefosse, where he did a research of aromatic oils and their ability to heal ailments. But the use of essential oils has long existed dating back to the 10th century when the Persians first invented the process of distillation. History suggests that aromatherapy has been used by European physicians about 2000 years ago.

Terms:

The first thing we need to do in order to understand fully this natural science is to know some of the different terminologies which are used in this industry.

* Essential oils- These oils are the also known as volatile oils, aetherolea, or any kind of oil extracted from a plant or herb. They are obtained through distillation and, in some researches, are called the "spirit" of the plant because it carries the characteristics of the plant itself. These oils, when inhaled or mixed in bathwater, produce a reaction

from the body depending on what type of fruit or herb the oil was extracted from.

* Aromatherapy- According to the Merriam-Webster dictionary, it is the process of massaging the body, especially the face, with a mixture of fragrant essential oils extracted from herbs, flowers, and fruits. Basically, it is promoting the well-being of the body through the massage of essential oils. This process is categorized in different types due to its many different uses which are clinical aromatherapy, essential oil therapy and aromatic medicine, amongst several.

* Distillation- The process of extracting gas or vapor from either solids or liquids through heating or cooling.

* Extraction- The act of removing or taking out something usually through a certain amount of force or an effort.

Chapter 2. Ways of Essential Oil Extraction

There are several ways in extracting essential oils and it usually depends highly on where you will extract them from but the ones below are the basic ones used even in ancient times and have just been improved and made easier over the course of time but are essentially the same in nature.

1. Steam Distillation - There are more than one way of steam distillation which are:

Water Distillation

Straight Steam Distillation

Water/Steam Distillation

a) Water Distillation- is the process where the plant or herb is boiled in water and the steam and oil coming from it will be separated to produce the essential oil.

b) Straight Steam Distillation- is where the plant material is pushed through with steam, therefore, capturing the essential oils in it.

c) Water/Steam Distillation- is the process of pushing through and around the plant material with steam and water to extract the essential oils.

2. Expression - Mostly used for extraction of citrus oils from fruits like lemon and lime with the use of a cooling method and not through the process of heating. Expressed oils are the ones taken from the fruit rinds and no heat is used in doing it.

3. Solvent Extraction - This process uses other materials such as hexane and acetone and other chemicals in extracting the essential oils. This is mainly what the perfume manufacturers practice because of the need of massively producing the perfumes in the fastest way possible in the most cost-efficient manner. The use of essential oils in perfumes have become very popular and widely used nowadays.

4. Enfleurage - is probably the oldest and now, the least type of method in extraction being used. It is the use of odorless animal fats to capture the fragrant oils of flowers and plants. It is a very tedious and expensive method because it involves the use of other

compounds like the animal fat and various steps to simply extract the oils.

5. Phytonic Process - it is the latest method of oil extraction which was developed in England in 1994 whereby it uses fluorocarbons in extracting the essential oils.

6. Carbon Dioxide Extraction- is the use of CO_2 in extraction of essential oils. This method proves to be safer to use than Solvent Extraction because CO_2 is non-toxic and non-flammable compared to hexane and acetone which are used in solvent extraction.

These are some of the more popular ways in extracting the essential oils in plants, flowers, and herbs but there might be other methods or variations of these methods found in different fields of essential oil manufacturing.

Chapter 3. Uses of Essential Oils

Just like the ways in extracting these essential oils, there are also many types of essential oils that are used in several ways like stress-relief, weight-loss, different types of massages, and many more. Let's enumerate these oils and how they are used by the body.

1. Weight-loss Essential Oils

Gaining too much is a world-wide problem for many and using organic and natural methods in losing weight has become the new trend nowadays because it is healthier and less dangerous to the person. In line with this, many have concocted a number of weight-loss essential oil mixtures promising great results in losing weight. These are some of the essential oils used to lose weight and how to make them.

a) Peppermint Essential Oils

This is recommended to curb your cravings and promote good digestion. Peppermint has a special quality that makes your brain think you're already full and participants in some researches in this type of weight-loss method have had fewer cravings and feel less hungry when they inhaled peppermint oils. This kind of plant is also full of nutrients like vitamin C, omega3 fatty acids, iron and magnesium just to name a few. This oil promotes a healthy way of losing those unwanted cravings therefore reducing your calorie content in a safe way.

Peppermint Essential Oils Recipe:

Here's a recipe of how to make Peppermint Essential Oil that everyone can enjoy and easily make.

Ingredients: Dried peppermint leaves, coffee filters or paper coffee filters, grain alcohol or vodka, a funnel, and two jars with one having a tight lid.

Steps:

Crush the dried peppermint leaves and put it in one jar. You can fill the whole jar with these crushed leaves for more uses.

Fill the jar with the grain alcohol or vodka. Do not use rubbing alcohol or isopropyl alcohol because it is not safe and will not bring out the desired effects.

Shake the jar several times a day so the oils can be released and continue doing so for three days in a row. Be careful not to store it longer because the concoction might go bad and will just ruin your efforts.

With the coffee filter, strain the liquid into the other jar and once filtered, just cover it with a clean cloth and let it sit for about week so the alcohol will evaporate leaving only the essential oils.

Strain it again to remove the sediments that might have formed and place the oil in a smaller jar, preferably a tinted one so the heat and sunlight won't degrade the quality of the peppermint oil.

There you go! You have successfully made a Peppermint Essential Oil extract which you can use in several ways to reduce your weight.

Uses:

Adding a few drops in your bath every morning will curb those cravings and jumpstart your day.

Diffusing a few drops to inhale before eating will help suppress your appetite.

You can also add a drop or two in your drink during meals to reduce your appetite.

b) Lemon Essential Oils

Lemons contain many vitamins and minerals that are good for the body like vitamin C and d-Limonene. This kind of essential oil helps in digestion and balancing metabolism and gives you the energy you need to go through your day. It helps address problems with intestinal parasites and other stomach ailments.

Lemon Essential Oil Recipe:

Ingredients: A lemon and a cold-pressed olive oil

Steps:

Grate the lemon skin and place in a bowl.

Fill half of a glass bottle with the grated lemon zest and half with the cold-pressed olive oil

Leave the bottle in a place with lots of sunlight, shaking it a few times a day for several days, around 3 days.

Once lemon oil is achieved, store in a place with room temperature.

Uses:

Inhale diffused lemon oil before meals.
For a detoxifying effect, add 1 or 2 drops of lemon essential oil in your drink before breakfast.
You can rub and massage this oil in areas where there is cellulite because it can help remove toxins that are stored in fat cells which will make your body thinner and healthier.

c) Grapefruit Essential Oils

Grapefruit is known to contain d-Limonene which helps release fatty acids into the bloodstream where it is broken down and finally used for energy. It contains vitamin C and Lycopene which is a powerful antioxidant which detoxifies and cleans the lymphatic system.

Grapefruit Essential Oils Recipe:

Ingredients: Grapefruit Rind, small spoon, kitchen grater, small crock pot, cheesecloth, dark bottle (including stopper), and almond oil.

Steps:

1. Grate the grapefruit peel or zest the grapefruit.

2. Place grapefruit rinds in a lean plate and set out to dry, It might a couple of days depending on the size of the rinds, the smaller they are, the quicker they will dry.

3. Place the lemon zest or rind into the crock pot and top it off with almond oil. Lower the heat of the crock pot to low and cover it. Let the mixture blend and heat for 8 hours.

4. Pour the oil from the crock pot into a bowl lined with five layers of cheesecloth. Position the cloth in a way that you can squeeze out all the oils into the bowl.

5. Pour the contents in small containers and seal with cork stoppers or lids. Store in a cool, dry place but do not refrigerate it.

Uses:

Add 1 or 2 drops of the grapefruit essential oil to your drinking water to flush out toxins and experience the fat burning effects. It is ideal to drink this before breakfast which also enhances the food flavor.

Massage into skin where there are cellulites by combining 1 to 2 drops of it with organic virgin coconut oil and don't wash off for a few hours.

You can also add 5 drops with a warm water bath and soak for about 30 minutes. You can combine other oils for better results of losing cellulite during bathing.

2. Stress-Relieving Essential Oils

Stress is an everyday effect of life. Whether we like it or not, we will get stressed every once in a while, some more that others, it depends on your career, family, and your social life as a whole. So one of the ways to fight off stress is by the use of essential oils to soothe the senses and relax the mind. Here are some essential oils that can be used to relieve stress anytime.

a) Lavender Essential Oils

It has a calming, lightly sweet fragrance that relaxes both the body and the emotions and can be used to relieve muscle pains and joint pains. It can also be used for minor cuts, burns and bug bites as an antiseptic.

Lavender Essential Oils Recipe:

Ingredients: container with a tight lid, carrier oil like olive oil, strainer or cheesecloth, dark glass bottle

Steps:

1. Pour lavender into a glass jar with the leaves already cut. Pour the carrier oil at least halfway the bottle container and let it sit for about 48 hours.

2. Shake the container periodically over the 48 hours to let the oils out. Make sure that you let it sit in a warm spot where there is lots of sun.

3. Strain the essential oils with the strainer or cheesecloth and put the contents in the dark glass bottle and put the lid on.

4. Store in a cool dry place which can last a year.

Uses:

Apply small amounts to the skin and the oil will penetrate through your skin into the bloodstream soothing stress and anxiety in the process.

Inhale a few drops of this lavender oil to relieve some of that stress.

b) Rose Essential Oils

Rose essential oils can relieve stress and depression as well as help in the healing of eczema and menopausal signs and symptoms. It might be costly because it takes around 60,000 roses just to get 1 ounce of rose oil.

Rose Essential Oils Recipe:

Ingredients: 4 cups of rose petals, 12 x 12 muslin cloth , rubber band, organic carrier oil(16oz), potato masher, and a gallon of mason jar

Steps:

1. Spread the 4 cups of rose petals with hips onto the muslin cloth.

2. Slowly wrap the rose petals and hips and secure the muslin cloth with rubber band, making sure the petals and hips don't fall out.

3. Drop the cloth into the mason jar.

4. Add the carrier oil with 16 oz.

5. Use the potato masher to mash the muslin cloth but not too much that it might puncture it. Continue mashing it in with the carrier oil and close the lid.

6. Store in a cool dry place for 2 weeks

7. Discard the rose petals and hips and replace with another batch of 4 cups. Repeat process for about 4-5 times.

Uses:

Diffuse oil and inhale whenever you want or whenever stressed. It will help relax your anxieties.

c) Chamomile Essential Oils

These are suited to calm the nerves and help in healthy digestion. There are two types of chamomile oils which are the Roman type and the German type. The Roman type is used more in mental anxiety, hostility and paranoia while the German type is used more for the treatment of irritated skin.

Chamomile Essential Oils Recipe: It is basically how the other essential oils are extracted. Refer to the recipe steps above.

Uses:

Known to relieve stress effectively through inhalation or diffusion into the air with the use of candles or by adding a few drops in candle wax oils.

3. Beauty Essential Oils

There are numerous essential oils that are great for skin rejuvenation and produce moisturizing effects. The recipes for these essential oils are basically the same as other essential oils are extracted.

a) Sesame Essential Oils

This oil is great with hair and skin remedies, it moisturizes the skin and has an SPF factor to shield the skin form harsh sunlight. The fatty acids in sesame oils are believed to lower stress as well as blood pressure and has been suggested to help slow down the growth of cancer cells in the body.

Uses:

Massage into skin and face after a hot bath and leave for 10 minutes. Wipe of oil with warm cloth. This will trap the moisture in your skin so it leaves it clean and moisturized for the whole day.

You can also use this as a natural sunscreen lotion because of its SPF factor. You can use it daily to keep your skin young and smooth-looking.

b) Rose Otto/ Rose Essential Oil

Apart from relieving stress and tension in the body, it also improves the look of your skin through its aromatic qualities.

Uses:

Add a few drops to your bath or mix it with other oils for better effect.

c) Geranium Essential Oils

Contains astringent properties which refreshes the skin and also has styptic effects which have medicinal effects as well. This multipurpose essential oil can be used for treating acne, reducing oily skin, improve blood circulation, and reduce acne scars. Geraniums also reduce the appearance of fine lines and wrinkles and can calm inflammations.

Uses:

You can directly inhale this essential oil to calm the senses and promote better health.

Apply several drops to the temples or abdomen for soothing purposes.

It may also be used as dietary supplement with just a few drops of this oil.

d) Carrot Seed Essential Oils

It rejuvenates the skin by helping it stay smooth and helps regenerate cells in the body. It's also proven to reduce scars and reduce skin aging by improving skin tone.

Uses:

Diffused, inhaled or adding a few drops to your drink for consumption will promote better skin qualities.

e) Lavender Essential Oils

It helps lighten age spots and scars that appear on the skin and also help in skin regeneration. It is great for all skin types especially for those who have mature skin, skin spots, and skin with scars.

Uses:

Can be diffused, inhaled or added to your everyday bath for better skin care.

4. Body Massage Essential Oils

Just like the essential oils in beauty care, essential oils are good for the entire body because is the most natural way of helping improve the condition of the body and its various parts and organs as well as the emotional well-being of a person. All the essentials oils mentioned above are good for the body. It will just depend on where and for what ailment you will be using these various essential oils. Essential oils used in massages will help the body's blood circulation, facilitate detoxification and draining of lymphocytes and many more.

There are many massage essential oils being used today namely:

Cel-Lite Magic Massage Oil- improves circulation by getting rid of lactic acid in the muscles which promotes healthy body functions. It detoxifies and cleans the skin all over and generally improves skin quality.

Dragon Time Massage Oil- is a blend of different oils that is designed for women to help ease the mind, mood changes, and cramps brought about by the menstrual cycle. There are six different oils used in dragon oil which are: Jasmine Absolute, Clary Sage Essential Oil, Marjoram Essential Oil, Lavender Essential Oil, Fennel Essential Oil, and Blue Yarrow Essential Oil.

Ortho Ease Massage Oil- is a mixture of various vegetable oils and essential oils that promote muscle relaxation and helps with minor pains and aches from extraneous activities. It also improves circulation of the body and flush out toxins energizing the person and increases body flexibility

Ortho Sport Massage Oil- for the more sporty body who likes to hit the gym several times a week, it is great to apply before and after working out to improve circulation and address minor aches and pains. When applied and massaged into skin, it loosens muscles and make them more flexible and less stiff for better body performance.

Relaxation Massage Oil- not only used to relieve the tension of the body from activities of the day, it also helps in soothing and calming the mind and emotional disposition and restore vigor. It is best to use this oil mixed with your hot bath before hitting the sack to you can relax your tense muscles and clear the mind for a good night's sleep.

Sensation Massage Oil- the functions are more of uplifting and arousing the senses. It is more of a perfume than oil but it is great to massage into your skin. There are three therapeutic grades for this essential oil which are: Ylang Ylang Essential Oil, Rosewood Essential Oil, and Jasmine Absolute.

V-6 Mixing Oil- this massage oil contains six vegetable oils which are coconut oils, grape seed oils, wheat germ oils, and, of course, olive oils.

Chapter 4. Benefits and Other Uses of Essential Oils

* Easy to use and ingredients are very easy to find. They are very convenient to have around because you can just inhale it, put a few drops in your drink or diffuse it. They can be carried everywhere, anytime. Plus if you want to make your own, it's fairly easy to do and you can find everything you need in the kitchen.

* Essential oils have oxygenating effects. They can transport nutrients, vitamins and minerals to the cells especially those that are oxygen- deprived.

* Essential oils are high in antioxidants. Antioxidants improve the quality of the skin and strengthen the body's immune system preventing aging, and other harmful effects of pollutants in the air.

* Essential oils sooth digestion. It may repair and restore digestive functions when taken, especially with Peppermint essential oils.

* Essential oils are organic or natural. It is the most organic oil that has medicinal and healing properties with little or no possible harmful side effects to the

body. Since the ingredients are mostly plants, herbs, flowers, and fruits and vegetables, no other chemicals are extracted which can be very toxic to the body.

* Essential oils can improve your outlook in life by helping reduce anxiety and depression b uplifting your spirits with just a sniff.

* Essential oils can be used by everybody and anybody. Even children can use essential oils, of course, you still need to make sure those you are using are safe enough and are in small amounts so as not to do more harm than good. The ones mostly used are chamomile and peppermint essential oils because they can be mixed in with teas or drinks to promote good sleep for children.

* Essential oils can also be used in the house. It's an alternative way of cleansing your house of impurities and germs. Now, you don't need to just rely on chemical-based air fresheners that might be toxic for you and your children.

* Essential oils can give you deep spiritual awareness. Since plants and flowers are used in religious and spiritual ceremonies, it activates the senses, as research shows, and stimulates olfactory receptors.

These essential oils in their pure constituents activate the limbic system which is associated with memory, emotion, and state of mind.

Final Words

Essential oils have been around since before spas and treatment centers were created and used for the general public's well-being and centers where you seek better health. The most basic of essential oils are very easy to cultivate and make that you can make your own version at home without spending so much on chemicals or other toxic concoctions that lead promise great results but not really deliver. With the different uses of essential oils in Aromatherapy and in our everyday lives, it's hard to think of it as having any negative effects to the body in general. However, all things must be used in moderation so keep in mind that even the use of essential oils must be regulated and still try to do you research and better yet, consult medical practitioners on which oils are safe enough to use daily.

Your health and well-being must be your utmost priority in all things you do. Do not abuse your body because you're young and can take all the stress and pressure from your work or your vices. Learn to use essential oils now in health ailments and minor home remedies and the results will satisfy you in the end.

There is no shortage of plants and herbs you can use for your essential oils and aromatherapy sessions to better pick up the habit and live healthier lifestyle with a positive outlook in life. Aromatherapy with the use of essential oils will get you there.

Thank You Page

I want to personally thank you for reading my book. I hope you found information in this book useful and I would be very grateful if you could leave your honest review about this book. I certainly want to thank you in advance for doing this.

CPSIA information can be obtained
at www.ICGtesting.com
Printed in the USA
BVHW041819030419

544511BV00020B/420/P